ANTI-INFLAMMAT ORY COOKBOOK FOR BEGINNERS:

300+ Delicious and Healthy Recipes for Beginners - Restore Your Body and Reduce Inflammation Effortlessly!

BY

NELSON ROBINSON

TABLE OF CONTENTS

INTRODUCTION..**4**

CHAPTER 1: ANTI-INFLAMMATORY BASICS....8

Understanding Inflammation and its Impact on Health...8

The Fundamentals of the Anti-Inflammatory Diet.. 14

Building a Foundation: Essential Ingredients and Kitchen Tools...20

CHAPTER 2: BREAKFAST DELIGHTS................ 26

Berry Blast Smoothie...26

Quinoa Breakfast Bowl... 28

Avocado Toast with Turmeric.................................30

Chia Seed Pudding with Mixed Berries.................. 32

Spinach and Mushroom Omelette........................... 34

Golden Milk Overnight Oats.................................. 36

CHAPTER 3: LUNCH FOR WELLNESS................ 38

Mediterranean Chickpea Salad................................38

Grilled Salmon with Citrus Glaze.......................... 40

Turmeric Chicken and Vegetable Wrap..................42

Lentil and Vegetable Stew...................................... 44

Quinoa and Kale Salad with Lemon Tahini Dressing. 46

Sweet Potato and Black Bean Buddha Bowl...........48

CHAPTER 4: DINNER FOR RENEWAL.................50

Baked Cod with Garlic and Herbs...........................50

Cauliflower Rice Stir-Fry..52

Tomato Basil Zoodle Bowl......................................54

Turmeric and Ginger Spiced Chicken......................56

Salmon and Asparagus Foil Pack............................58

Butternut Squash and Lentil Curry..........................60

Chapter 5: Snacking Smart......................................62

Almond and Turmeric Energy Bites........................62

Greek Yogurt Parfait with Berries and Nuts............64

Roasted Chickpeas with Smoky Paprika..................66

Veggie Sticks with Hummus....................................68

Trail Mix with Anti-Inflammatory Spices...............70

Cucumber Avocado Salsa..72

CONCLUSION...74

INTRODUCTION

In a world where fast-paced lifestyles often dictate our dietary choices, the importance of maintaining a healthy, inflammation-free body cannot be overstated. As we usher in 2024, the need for comprehensive well-being takes center stage, and what better way to start than by embracing the transformative power of an anti-inflammatory diet?

Welcome to "Nourish and Thrive: An Anti-Inflammatory Cookbook for Beginners 2024." This cookbook is not just a collection of recipes; it's a guide to a lifestyle that promotes optimal health and vitality. Inflammation, the body's natural response to injury or infection, can become chronic when triggered by factors like stress, poor dietary choices, and environmental toxins. This chronic inflammation has been linked to a myriad of health issues, from arthritis and digestive disorders to cardiovascular diseases and even certain cancers.

Our cookbook is designed for those who are ready to embark on a journey toward a healthier, more balanced life. Whether you're a novice in the kitchen or a seasoned chef, our carefully curated recipes cater to all skill levels, making the transition to an anti-inflammatory diet both accessible and delicious.

In the pages that follow, you'll discover a treasure trove of recipes crafted to soothe inflammation and promote overall wellness. From vibrant salads bursting with nutrient-rich ingredients to hearty one-pot wonders that simplify mealtime, each dish is thoughtfully created to not only tantalize your taste buds but also nourish your body from the inside out.

But this cookbook is more than just a compilation of recipes; it's an educational tool. We'll delve into the science behind inflammation, exploring the powerful impact that food choices can have on our bodies. With a deeper understanding of the relationship between diet and inflammation, you'll be empowered to make informed choices that support your well-being.

As you embark on this culinary journey, envision a life where every meal is an opportunity to nurture your body and celebrate the incredible flavors that nature provides.

"Nourish and Thrive: An Anti-Inflammatory Cookbook for Beginners 2024" is your roadmap to a healthier, more vibrant you. Let the adventure begin!

CHAPTER 1: ANTI-INFLAMMATOR Y BASICS

Understanding Inflammation and its Impact on Health

Inflammation is a natural and essential part of the body's defense mechanism, playing a crucial role in the healing process. However, when inflammation becomes chronic, it can contribute to various health issues. Understanding the basics of inflammation and adopting anti-inflammatory practices is essential for maintaining overall well-being.

What is Inflammation?

Inflammation is the body's response to injury, infection, or harmful stimuli. It is a complex biological process that involves the immune system, blood vessels, and various signaling molecules. The purpose of inflammation is to eliminate the cause of cell injury, clear out damaged cells and tissues, and initiate tissue repair.

Acute vs. Chronic Inflammation:

1. Acute Inflammation:

Rapid onset and short duration.

Typically a protective and localized response.

Examples include a cut, infection, or injury.

2. Chronic Inflammation:

Long-term, persistent inflammation.

Can contribute to various diseases, such as arthritis, cardiovascular diseases, and autoimmune disorders.

Often associated with lifestyle factors like poor diet, stress, and lack of exercise.

The Link Between Inflammation and Health:
Chronic inflammation is increasingly recognized as a contributing factor to many health conditions. Conditions linked to chronic

inflammation include:
1. *Cardiovascular diseases*
2. *Diabetes*
3. *Autoimmune disorders*
4. *Neurodegenerative diseases*
5. *Certain cancers*

Anti-Inflammatory Lifestyle:
Adopting an anti-inflammatory lifestyle can help manage chronic inflammation and promote overall health. Key components include:

1. Healthy Diet:

Emphasize whole, nutrient-dense foods.

Include anti-inflammatory foods such as fatty fish, fruits, vegetables, nuts, and seeds.

Limit or avoid processed foods, refined sugars, and trans fats.

2. Regular Exercise:

Promotes circulation and reduces inflammation.

Engage in a mix of aerobic and strength-training exercises.

3. Stress Management:

Chronic stress can contribute to inflammation.

Practice relaxation techniques such as meditation, yoga, or deep breathing.

4. Quality Sleep:

Inadequate sleep may promote inflammation.

Aim for 7-9 hours of quality sleep per night.

5. Hydration:

Water is essential for overall health and can help flush out toxins.

Anti-Inflammatory Supplements:

Certain supplements may have anti-inflammatory properties, including:

1. *Omega-3 fatty acids*
2. *Turmeric and curcumin*
3. *Ginger*
4. *Vitamin D*
5. *Probiotics*

It's important to consult with a healthcare professional before incorporating supplements into your routine.

Understanding the basics of inflammation and its impact on health is crucial for adopting a proactive approach to well-being. By incorporating anti-inflammatory practices into your lifestyle, such as a healthy diet, regular exercise, stress management, and adequate sleep, you can contribute to reducing the risk of chronic inflammation and promoting overall health. Always consult with healthcare professionals for personalized advice and guidance on managing inflammation.

The Fundamentals of the Anti-Inflammatory Diet

In recent years, the importance of maintaining an anti-inflammatory lifestyle has gained significant attention in the realm of health and wellness. Chronic inflammation has been linked to a variety of health issues, including heart disease, diabetes, and autoimmune disorders. One effective way to combat inflammation is through adopting an anti-inflammatory diet. In this article, we will explore the fundamentals of the anti-inflammatory diet and how incorporating certain foods can promote overall well-being.

Understanding Inflammation:

Before delving into the anti-inflammatory diet, it's crucial to understand inflammation itself. Inflammation is a natural response of the body to injury or infection, but when it becomes chronic, it can lead to long-term health problems. The anti-inflammatory diet focuses on reducing inflammation by incorporating foods that have been shown to have anti-inflammatory properties.

Key Components of the Anti-Inflammatory Diet:

Fruits and Vegetables:

Rich in antioxidants, vitamins, and minerals, fruits and vegetables play a pivotal role in an anti-inflammatory diet. Berries, leafy greens, and colorful vegetables are particularly high in anti-inflammatory compounds.

Healthy Fats:

Omega-3 fatty acids, found in fatty fish like salmon, flaxseeds, chia seeds, and walnuts, have potent anti-inflammatory effects. Additionally, extra virgin olive oil is an excellent source of monounsaturated fats with anti-inflammatory properties.

Whole Grains:

Opt for whole grains like brown rice, quinoa, and oats instead of refined grains. Whole grains contain fiber and nutrients that contribute to a balanced and anti-inflammatory diet.

Lean Proteins:

Choose lean protein sources such as poultry, fish, tofu, and legumes. These foods provide essential amino acids without the inflammatory effects associated with some red meats.

Herbs and Spices:

Many herbs and spices have anti-inflammatory properties. Turmeric, ginger, garlic, and cinnamon are known for their ability to reduce inflammation and contribute flavor to your meals.

Nuts and Seeds:

Almonds, walnuts, and flaxseeds are rich in omega-3 fatty acids and antioxidants. These can be great additions to snacks or meals to enhance the anti-inflammatory aspect of your diet.

Probiotics:

Fermented foods like yogurt, kefir, and sauerkraut contain probiotics that support gut health. A healthy gut microbiome is linked to reduced inflammation throughout the body.

Limit Processed Foods:
Processed foods, high in trans fats and refined sugars, can contribute to inflammation. Minimize the intake of these foods and focus on whole, nutrient-dense options.

Adopting an anti-inflammatory diet is a proactive and holistic approach to promoting overall health and well-being. By incorporating a variety of nutrient-dense foods rich in antioxidants, omega-3 fatty acids, and other anti-inflammatory compounds, you can support your body in its fight against chronic inflammation. Remember, consistency is key, and making small, sustainable changes to your diet can have a profound impact on your long-term health. Consult with a healthcare professional or a registered dietitian to tailor an anti-inflammatory diet that suits your individual needs and health goals.

Building a Foundation: Essential Ingredients and Kitchen Tools

Inflammation is a natural response of the body to injury or infection, but chronic inflammation can lead to various health issues. Adopting an anti-inflammatory lifestyle through proper nutrition is a powerful way to support overall well-being. In this guide, we'll explore the foundational elements of an anti-inflammatory diet, focusing on essential ingredients and kitchen tools that can make a significant difference in your journey to better health.

Essential Ingredients:

Fruits and Vegetables:

Rich in antioxidants and phytochemicals, fruits and vegetables play a crucial role in reducing inflammation. Berries, leafy greens, cruciferous vegetables, and colorful produce should be staples in an anti-inflammatory diet.

Fatty Fish:

Cold-water fish like salmon, mackerel, and sardines are high in omega-3 fatty acids, which have potent anti-inflammatory properties. Incorporating these into your diet can help balance the omega-3 to omega-6 ratio, a key factor in inflammation control.

Whole Grains:

Opt for whole grains such as quinoa, brown rice, and oats. These grains contain fiber and other nutrients that contribute to a healthy gut microbiome, which is linked to reduced inflammation.

Healthy Fats:

Include sources of healthy fats like avocados, olive oil, and nuts. These fats contain monounsaturated and polyunsaturated fats, which have anti-inflammatory effects.

Herbs and Spices:

Turmeric, ginger, garlic, and cinnamon are known for their anti-inflammatory properties. Incorporating these herbs and spices into your cooking not only enhances flavor but also boosts the nutritional value of your meals.

Kitchen Tools for an Anti-Inflammatory Kitchen:

High-Quality Blender:

A powerful blender is essential for preparing smoothies and soups with nutrient-dense ingredients. This tool allows you to easily incorporate a variety of fruits, vegetables, and herbs into your daily diet.

Steamer Basket:

Steaming is a gentle cooking method that helps retain the nutritional content of vegetables. A steamer basket is a versatile tool for cooking a variety of anti-inflammatory vegetables while preserving their health benefits.

Quality Knives and Cutting Boards:

Efficiently preparing fruits, vegetables, and lean proteins requires sharp knives and a durable cutting board. Investing in high-quality kitchen tools can make meal preparation more enjoyable and time-efficient.

Non-Stick Cookware:

Using non-stick cookware reduces the need for excessive cooking oils, promoting a heart-healthy and anti-inflammatory approach to cooking.

Food Processor:

A food processor is invaluable for chopping, slicing, and grinding ingredients. It simplifies the preparation of homemade dips, sauces, and nut-based recipes that are rich in anti-inflammatory nutrients.

Building a foundation for an anti-inflammatory lifestyle begins in the kitchen. By incorporating essential ingredients and utilizing the right tools, you can create delicious, nutritious meals that actively support your body's fight against inflammation. Embracing these basics not only enhances your overall well-being but also makes the journey towards an anti-inflammatory lifestyle both sustainable and enjoyable.

CHAPTER 2: BREAKFAST DELIGHTS

Berry Blast Smoothie

Time Frame: 5 minutes

Ingredients:

1. *1 cup mixed berries (strawberries, blueberries, raspberries)*
2. *1 banana*
3. *1/2 cup Greek yogurt*
4. *1/2 cup almond milk*
5. *1 tablespoon honey*
6. *Ice cubes (optional)*

Instructions:

1. *Combine all ingredients in a blender.*

2. *Blend until smooth and creamy.*

3. *Pour into a glass and enjoy your refreshing Berry Blast Smoothie!*

Tip:

1. *Add a handful of spinach for an extra nutrient boost without altering the taste.*

Quinoa Breakfast Bowl

Time Frame: 15 minutes

Ingredients:

1. *1 cup cooked quinoa*
2. *1/2 cup Greek yogurt*
3. *1/4 cup sliced almonds*
4. *1/2 cup mixed berries*
5. *1 tablespoon honey*

Instructions:

1. *In a bowl, layer quinoa and Greek yogurt.*
2. *Top with sliced almonds and mixed berries.*
3. *Drizzle honey over the bowl.*
4. *Mix before eating for a delicious and nutritious breakfast!*

Tip:

1. *Experiment with different fruits and nuts for variety.*

Avocado Toast with Turmeric

Time Frame: 10 minutes

Ingredients:

1. *2 slices whole-grain bread*
2. *1 ripe avocado*
3. *1 teaspoon turmeric powder*
4. *Salt and pepper to taste*
5. *Red pepper flakes (optional)*

Instructions:

1. *Toast the bread slices.*
2. *Mash the avocado and spread it evenly on the toast.*
3. *Sprinkle turmeric, salt, and pepper.*
4. *Add a dash of red pepper flakes for a kick.*

Tip:

1. *Add a poached or fried egg on top for extra protein.*

Chia Seed Pudding with Mixed Berries

Time Frame: 4 hours (for chilling)

Ingredients:

1. *1/4 cup chia seeds*
2. *1 cup almond milk*
3. *1 tablespoon honey*
4. *1/2 teaspoon vanilla extract*
5. *Mixed berries for topping*

Instructions:

1. *Mix chia seeds, almond milk, honey, and vanilla in a jar.*
2. *Refrigerate for at least 4 hours or overnight.*
3. *Top with mixed berries before serving.*

Tip:

1. *Prepare it the night before for a quick grab-and-go breakfast.*

Spinach and Mushroom Omelette

Time Frame: 15 minutes

Ingredients:

1. *3 eggs*
2. *Handful of fresh spinach*
3. *1/2 cup sliced mushrooms*
4. *Salt and pepper to taste*
5. *1 tablespoon olive oil*
6. *Grated cheese (optional)*

Instructions:

1. *Beat eggs in a bowl and season with salt and pepper.*
2. *Sauté spinach and mushrooms in olive oil until wilted.*

3. *Pour eggs over the veggies and cook until set.*

4. *Fold the omelette and sprinkle with cheese if desired.*

Tip:

1. *Customize with your favorite veggies for a personalized touch.*

Golden Milk Overnight Oats

Time Frame: 8 hours (overnight)

Ingredients:

1. *1/2 cup rolled oats*
2. *1/2 cup almond milk*
3. *1/2 teaspoon turmeric powder*
4. *1/4 teaspoon cinnamon*
5. *1 tablespoon honey*
6. *Chopped nuts for topping*

Instructions:

1. *Mix oats, almond milk, turmeric, cinnamon, and honey in a jar.*
2. *Refrigerate overnight.*
3. *Top with chopped nuts before serving.*

Tip:

1. *Add a pinch of black pepper to enhance turmeric absorption.*

CHAPTER 3: LUNCH FOR WELLNESS

Mediterranean Chickpea Salad

Time Frame:

Prep Time: 15 minutes

Cooking Time: 0 minutes

Total Time: 15 minutes

Ingredients:

1. *2 cans chickpeas, drained and rinsed*

2. *1 cucumber, diced*

3. *1 cup cherry tomatoes, halved*

4. *1/2 red onion, finely chopped*

5. *1/2 cup Kalamata olives, sliced*

6. *Feta cheese, crumbled*

7. *Fresh parsley, chopped*

Instructions:

1. *In a large bowl, combine chickpeas, cucumber, tomatoes, red onion, and olives.*

2. *Sprinkle feta cheese and parsley over the salad.*

3. *Toss the ingredients gently to combine.*

4. *Drizzle with olive oil and lemon juice.*

5. *Season with salt and pepper to taste.*

Tip:

1. *Let the salad marinate in the fridge for at least 30 minutes before serving to enhance the flavors.*

Grilled Salmon with Citrus Glaze

Time Frame:

Prep Time: 10 minutes

Cooking Time: 10 minutes

Total Time: 20 minutes

Ingredients:

1. *Salmon fillets*
2. *1/4 cup orange juice*
3. *2 tablespoons soy sauce*
4. *1 tablespoon honey*
5. *1 teaspoon grated ginger*
6. *1 clove garlic, minced*
7. *Salt and pepper*

Instructions:

1. *Preheat the grill to medium-high heat.*
2. *In a bowl, whisk together orange juice, soy sauce, honey, ginger, and garlic to make the glaze.*
3. *Season salmon with salt and pepper.*
4. *Grill salmon for about 4-5 minutes per side, basting with the citrus glaze.*
5. *Serve the grilled salmon with extra glaze.*

Tip:

1. *For extra flavor, let the salmon marinate in the glaze for 30 minutes before grilling.*

Turmeric Chicken and Vegetable Wrap

Time Frame:

Prep Time: 15 minutes

Cooking Time: 15 minutes

Total Time: 30 minutes

Ingredients:

1. *Chicken breast, thinly sliced*

2. *1 teaspoon turmeric powder*

3. *1 teaspoon cumin*

4. *1 teaspoon paprika*

5. *Tortillas*

6. *Hummus*

7. *Mixed vegetables (bell peppers, onions, zucchini), sliced*

Instructions:

1. *Mix turmeric, cumin, and paprika. Coat chicken slices with the spice mix.*
2. *Sauté chicken in a pan until cooked through.*
3. *In the same pan, sauté mixed vegetables until tender.*
4. *Warm tortillas and spread hummus on each.*
5. *Fill tortillas with the turmeric chicken and sautéed vegetables.*

Tip:

1. *Add a dollop of Greek yogurt or tzatziki for a cool and creamy element.*

Lentil and Vegetable Stew

Time Frame:

Prep Time: 15 minutes

Cooking Time: 30 minutes

Total Time: 45 minutes

Ingredients:

1. *1 cup dried lentils*
2. *1 onion, chopped*
3. *2 carrots, diced*
4. *2 celery stalks, sliced*
5. *3 cloves garlic, minced*
6. *1 can diced tomatoes*
7. *Vegetable broth*
8. *1 teaspoon cumin*
9. *1 teaspoon thyme*
10. *Salt and pepper*

Instructions:

1. *Rinse lentils and set aside.*

2. *Sauté onions, carrots, celery, and garlic in a pot until softened.*

3. *Add lentils, diced tomatoes, vegetable broth, cumin, thyme, salt, and pepper.*

4. *Bring to a boil, then simmer for 25-30 minutes.*

5. *Adjust seasoning before serving.*

Tip:

1. *Serve with crusty bread for a complete meal.*

Quinoa and Kale Salad with Lemon Tahini Dressing

Time Frame:

Prep Time: 20 minutes

Cooking Time: 15 minutes

Total Time: 35 minutes

Ingredients:

1. *1 cup quinoa*

2. *Kale, chopped*

3. *Cherry tomatoes, halved*

4. *Cucumber, diced*

5. *Red bell pepper, chopped*

6. *Feta cheese, crumbled*

7. *Lemon Tahini Dressing:*

8. *1/4 cup tahini*

9. *2 tablespoons olive oil*

10. *2 tablespoons lemon juice*

11. *1 clove garlic, minced*

12. *Salt and pepper*

Instructions:

1. *Cook quinoa according to package instructions.*

2. *In a large bowl, combine quinoa, kale, tomatoes, cucumber, bell pepper, and feta.*

3. *In a separate bowl, whisk together tahini, olive oil, lemon juice, garlic, salt, and pepper.*

4. *Drizzle dressing over the salad and toss to combine.*

Tip:

1. *Make extra dressing and store it separately for a quick and refreshing dressing throughout the week.*

Sweet Potato and Black Bean Buddha Bowl

Time Frame:

Prep Time: 15 minutes

Cooking Time: 25 minutes

Total Time: 40 minutes

Ingredients:

1. Sweet potatoes, diced

2. Black beans, cooked

3. Avocado, sliced

4. Quinoa, cooked

5. Cherry tomatoes, halved

6. Cilantro, chopped

Instructions:

1. *Roast sweet potatoes in the oven until tender.*

2. *Assemble bowls with quinoa, black beans, roasted sweet potatoes, avocado, tomatoes, and cilantro.*

Tip:

1. *Drizzle with a lime vinaigrette for a burst of freshness.*

2. *Feel free to adjust quantities and ingredients based on your preferences and dietary needs!*

CHAPTER 4: DINNER FOR RENEWAL

Baked Cod with Garlic and Herbs

Time Frame:

Prep Time: 10 minutes

Cooking Time: 15 minutes

Total Time: 25 minutes

Ingredients:

1. *Cod fillets*

2. *2 tablespoons olive oil*

3. *3 cloves garlic, minced*

4. *Fresh herbs (parsley, dill, or thyme)*

5. *Lemon slices*

6. *Salt and pepper*

Instructions:

1. *Preheat the oven to 400°F (200°C).*
2. *Place cod fillets on a baking sheet.*
3. *In a small bowl, mix olive oil, minced garlic, chopped herbs, salt, and pepper.*
4. *Brush the cod fillets with the garlic and herb mixture.*
5. *Top with lemon slices.*
6. *Bake for 15 minutes or until the fish flakes easily.*

Tip:

1. *Serve with a side of steamed vegetables or a light salad.*

Cauliflower Rice Stir-Fry

Time Frame:

Prep Time: 15 minutes

Cooking Time: 15 minutes

Total Time: 30 minutes

Ingredients:

1. *Cauliflower, riced*
2. *Mixed vegetables (bell peppers, broccoli, carrots)*
3. *2 tablespoons soy sauce*
4. *1 tablespoon sesame oil*
5. *Garlic, minced*
6. *Green onions, chopped*

Instructions:

1. *Stir-fry cauliflower rice and mixed vegetables in a pan over medium heat.*

2. *In a small bowl, mix soy sauce, sesame oil, and minced garlic.*

3. *Pour the sauce over the cauliflower rice and vegetables.*

4. *Cook for an additional 5-7 minutes.*

5. *Top with chopped green onions before serving.*

Tip:

1. *Add a protein of your choice like tofu, chicken, or shrimp for a complete meal.*

Tomato Basil Zoodle Bowl

Time Frame:

Prep Time: 10 minutes

Cooking Time: 10 minutes

Total Time: 20 minutes

Ingredients:

1. *Zucchini, spiralized (zoodles)*
2. *Cherry tomatoes, halved*
3. *Fresh basil, chopped*
4. *Olive oil*
5. *Parmesan cheese, grated*
6. *Salt and pepper*

Instructions:

1. *In a pan, sauté zoodles and cherry tomatoes in olive oil until tender.*

2. *Toss in chopped fresh basil and season with salt and pepper.*

3. *Serve in bowls and top with grated Parmesan cheese.*

Tip:

1. *Add grilled chicken or shrimp for extra protein.*

Turmeric and Ginger Spiced Chicken

Time Frame:

Prep Time: 15 minutes

Cooking Time: 20 minutes

Total Time: 35 minutes

Ingredients:

1. *Chicken breasts, sliced*

2. *1 teaspoon turmeric*

3. *1 teaspoon ground ginger*

4. *2 tablespoons olive oil*

5. *1 onion, chopped*

6. *Garlic, minced*

7. *Coconut milk*

8. *Salt and pepper*

Instructions:

1. *Season chicken slices with turmeric and ground ginger.*
2. *In a pan, heat olive oil and sauté chopped onion and garlic until softened.*
3. *Add chicken slices and cook until browned.*
4. *Pour in coconut milk and simmer until the chicken is cooked through.*
5. *Season with salt and pepper.*

Tip:

1. *Serve over brown rice or quinoa for a wholesome meal.*

Salmon and Asparagus Foil Pack

Time Frame:

Prep Time: 10 minutes

Cooking Time: 20 minutes

Total Time: 30 minutes

Ingredients:

1. *Salmon fillets*

2. *Asparagus spears*

3. *Lemon slices*

4. *2 tablespoons olive oil*

5. *Garlic powder*

6. *Dill, chopped*

7. *Salt and pepper*

Instructions:

1. Preheat the oven to 400°F (200°C).
2. Place salmon fillets and asparagus spears on a large sheet of foil.
3. Drizzle with olive oil and sprinkle with garlic powder, chopped dill, salt, and pepper.
4. Top with lemon slices.
5. Seal the foil to create a packet and bake for 20 minutes.

Tip:

1. Serve with a side of quinoa or couscous.

Butternut Squash and Lentil Curry

Time Frame:

Prep Time: 20 minutes

Cooking Time: 30 minutes

Total Time: 50 minutes

Ingredients:

1. *Butternut squash, cubed*
2. *Lentils*
3. *Coconut milk*
4. *Curry powder*
5. *Onion, chopped*
6. *Garlic, minced*
7. *Ginger, grated*
8. *Fresh cilantro, chopped*

Instructions:

1. *In a pot, sauté chopped onion, garlic, and grated ginger until fragrant.*
2. *Add curry powder and stir.*
3. *Add cubed butternut squash, lentils, and coconut milk.*
4. *Simmer until the squash and lentils are tender.*
5. *Garnish with fresh cilantro before serving.*

Tip:

1. *Serve over brown rice or with naan bread.*
2. *Feel free to customize these recipes based on your taste preferences and dietary needs!*

Chapter 5: Snacking Smart

Almond and Turmeric Energy Bites

Time Frame:

Prep Time: 15 minutes

Chilling Time: 30 minutes

Total Time: 45 minutes

Ingredients:

1. *1 cup rolled oats*

2. *1/2 cup almond butter*

3. *1/3 cup honey or maple syrup*

4. *1/2 cup ground almonds*

5. *1 teaspoon turmeric*

6. *1/2 teaspoon vanilla extract*

7. *Pinch of salt*

8. *Shredded coconut (optional, for coating)*

Instructions:

1. *In a bowl, mix rolled oats, almond butter, honey, ground almonds, turmeric, vanilla extract, and a pinch of salt.*

2. *Refrigerate the mixture for about 30 minutes.*

3. *Roll the chilled mixture into small balls.*

4. *Optional: Roll the energy bites in shredded coconut.*

5. *Store in the refrigerator.*

Tip:

1. *These energy bites are a great make-ahead snack for a quick energy boost.*

Greek Yogurt Parfait with Berries and Nuts

Time Frame:

Prep Time: 10 minutes

Total Time: 10 minutes

Ingredients:

1. *Greek yogurt*

2. *Mixed berries (strawberries, blueberries, raspberries)*

3. *Nuts (almonds, walnuts)*

4. *Honey*

Instructions:

1. *In a glass or bowl, layer Greek yogurt.*

2. *Add a layer of mixed berries and a sprinkle of nuts.*

3. *Repeat the layers.*

4. *Drizzle honey on top.*

Tip:

1. *Customize with your favorite fruits and nuts for variety.*

Roasted Chickpeas with Smoky Paprika

Time Frame:

Prep Time: 10 minutes

Roasting Time: 30 minutes

Total Time: 40 minutes

Ingredients:

1. *2 cans chickpeas, drained and rinsed*

2. *2 tablespoons olive oil*

3. *1 teaspoon smoked paprika*

4. *1/2 teaspoon cumin*

5. *Salt and pepper to taste*

Instructions:

1. *Preheat the oven to 400°F (200°C).*

2. *In a bowl, toss chickpeas with olive oil, smoked paprika, cumin, salt, and pepper.*

3. *Spread the chickpeas on a baking sheet.*

4. *Roast for about 30 minutes or until crispy, shaking the pan occasionally.*

Tip:

1. *These make a crunchy, protein-packed snack. Experiment with different spice combinations.*

Veggie Sticks with Hummus

Time Frame:

Prep Time: 15 minutes

Total Time: 15 minutes

Ingredients:

1. *Carrot sticks*

2. *Cucumber sticks*

3. *Bell pepper strips*

4. *Cherry tomatoes*

5. *Hummus*

Instructions:

1. *Wash and cut veggies into sticks or strips.*

2. Arrange on a plate.

3. Serve with a bowl of hummus for dipping.

Tip:

1. Prepare extra veggies for a quick and healthy snack throughout the week.

Trail Mix with Anti-Inflammatory Spices

Time Frame:

Prep Time: 5 minutes

Total Time: 5 minutes

Ingredients:

1. *Mixed nuts (almonds, walnuts, cashews)*

2. *Dried fruits (cranberries, raisins)*

3. *Pumpkin seeds*

4. *1 teaspoon ground cinnamon*

5. *1/2 teaspoon turmeric*

6. *Pinch of black pepper*

Instructions:

1. *In a bowl, mix mixed nuts, dried fruits, and pumpkin seeds.*
2. *Sprinkle ground cinnamon, turmeric, and black pepper over the mix.*
3. *Toss to combine.*

Tip:

1. *The anti-inflammatory spices add flavor and health benefits to this classic snack.*

Cucumber Avocado Salsa

Time Frame:

Prep Time: 15 minutes

Total Time: 15 minutes

Ingredients:

1. *2 cucumbers, diced*

2. *2 avocados, diced*

3. *1 cup cherry tomatoes, halved*

4. *1/4 cup red onion, finely chopped*

5. *1/4 cup cilantro, chopped*

6. *Lime juice*

7. *Salt and pepper to taste*

Instructions:

1. *In a bowl, combine diced cucumbers, avocados, cherry tomatoes, red onion, and cilantro.*

2. *Squeeze fresh lime juice over the mixture.*

3. *Season with salt and pepper.*

4. *Gently toss to combine.*

Tip:

1. *Serve with whole-grain chips or use it as a topping for grilled chicken or fish.*

CONCLUSION

In conclusion, the "Anti-Inflammatory Cookbook for Beginners 2024: The Ultimate Step-by-Step Guide Beginner's Guide to the Anti-Inflammatory Diet with a Full-Color Cookbook to Enhance the Immune System & Reduce Inflammation" is a comprehensive and invaluable resource for anyone seeking to take charge of their health and well-being. Authored with precision and expertise, this book not only provides a thorough understanding of the principles behind the anti-inflammatory diet but also equips readers with practical tools to seamlessly incorporate these principles into their daily lives.

One of the standout features of this cookbook is its accessibility, making the anti-inflammatory diet approachable for beginners. The step-by-step guide simplifies the process of transitioning to an anti-inflammatory lifestyle, offering clear explanations and actionable tips. The inclusion of a full-color cookbook adds a delightful visual component to the experience, making the journey towards a healthier lifestyle not only educational but also visually appealing.

The authors demonstrate a deep understanding of the science behind inflammation and its impact on the body. They skillfully navigate complex nutritional concepts, presenting them in a way that is easy for readers to comprehend. By emphasizing the connection between diet and inflammation, the book empowers individuals to make informed choices that can lead to a reduction in inflammation and an enhancement of the immune system.

Moreover, the recipes featured in the cookbook are not only health-conscious but also delicious, proving that adopting an anti-inflammatory diet does not mean sacrificing flavor. From vibrant salads to hearty main courses, each recipe is thoughtfully crafted to maximize nutritional benefits without compromising taste. The inclusion of a full-color cookbook not only enhances the visual appeal of the recipes but also serves as a practical guide for preparing nutritious and satisfying meals.

Beyond the recipes, the book delves into the broader implications of an anti-inflammatory lifestyle, exploring its potential to address various health concerns. It emphasizes the role of food as medicine, highlighting how dietary choices can positively impact conditions ranging from arthritis to cardiovascular health. This holistic approach sets the book apart, providing readers with a comprehensive understanding of the far-reaching benefits of adopting an anti-inflammatory diet.

In the rapidly evolving landscape of health and wellness, the "Anti-Inflammatory Cookbook for Beginners 2024" stands out as a timely and indispensable guide. By merging scientific knowledge with practical advice and mouthwatering recipes, the authors have created a resource that not only educates but also inspires. Whether you are a newcomer to the anti-inflammatory diet or a seasoned practitioner looking for fresh insights, this book is a must-read that will undoubtedly leave a lasting impact on your journey towards a healthier and more vibrant life.